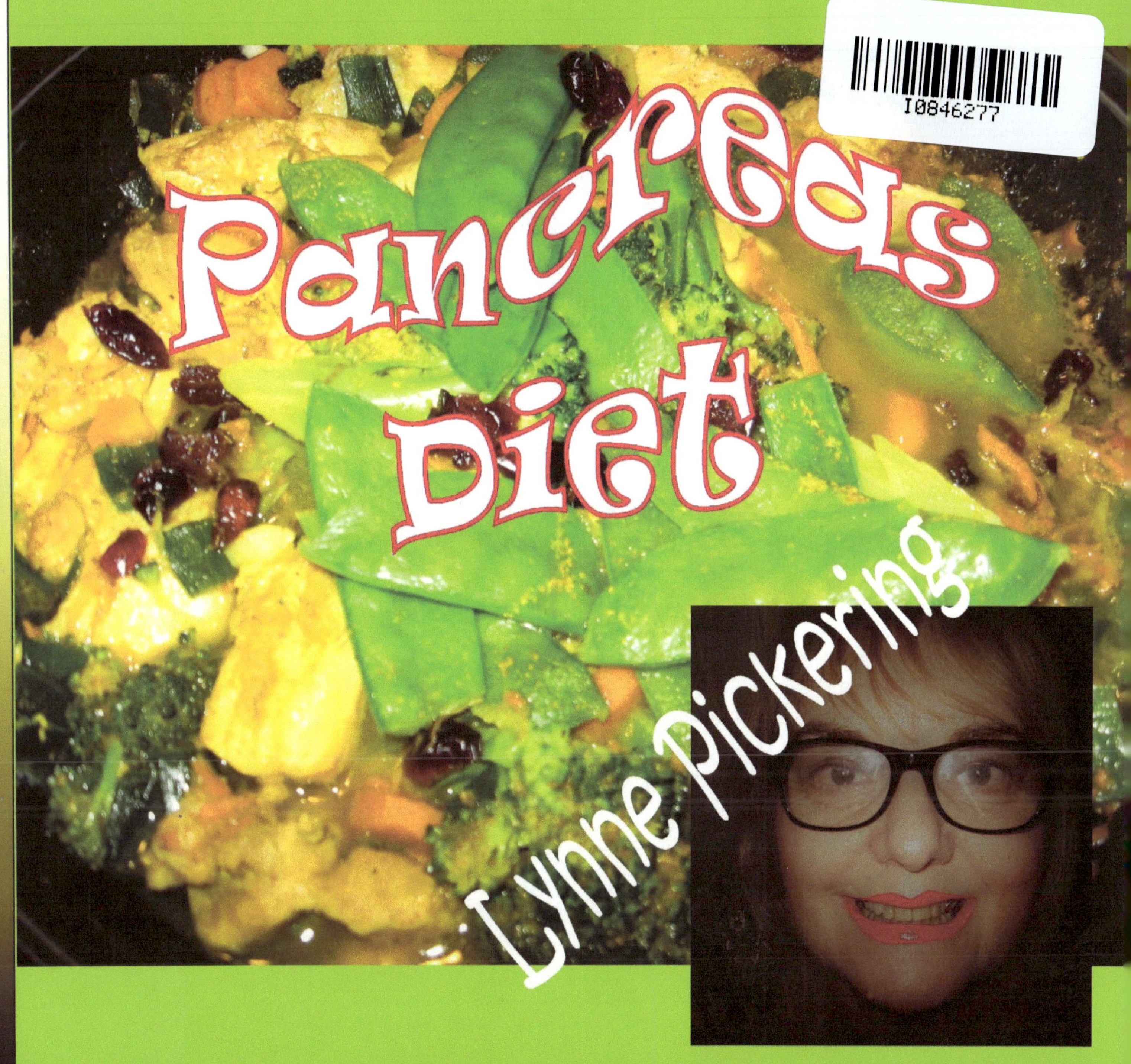

Pancreas Diet
Lynne Pickering

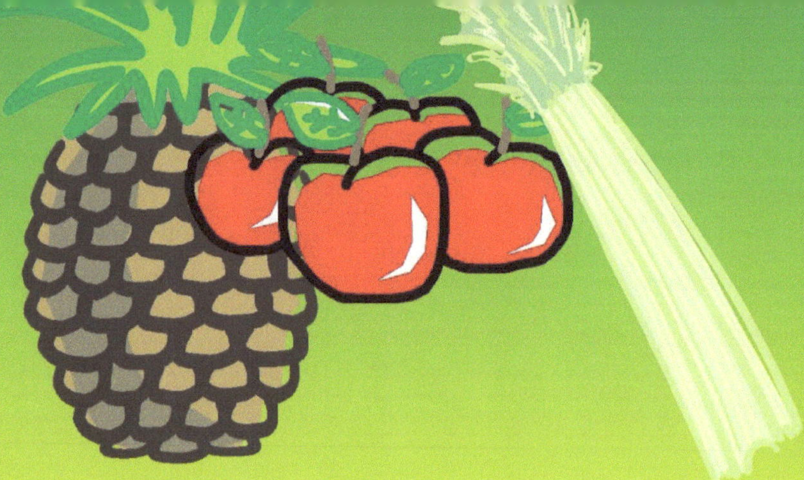

ISBN   978-1689870306

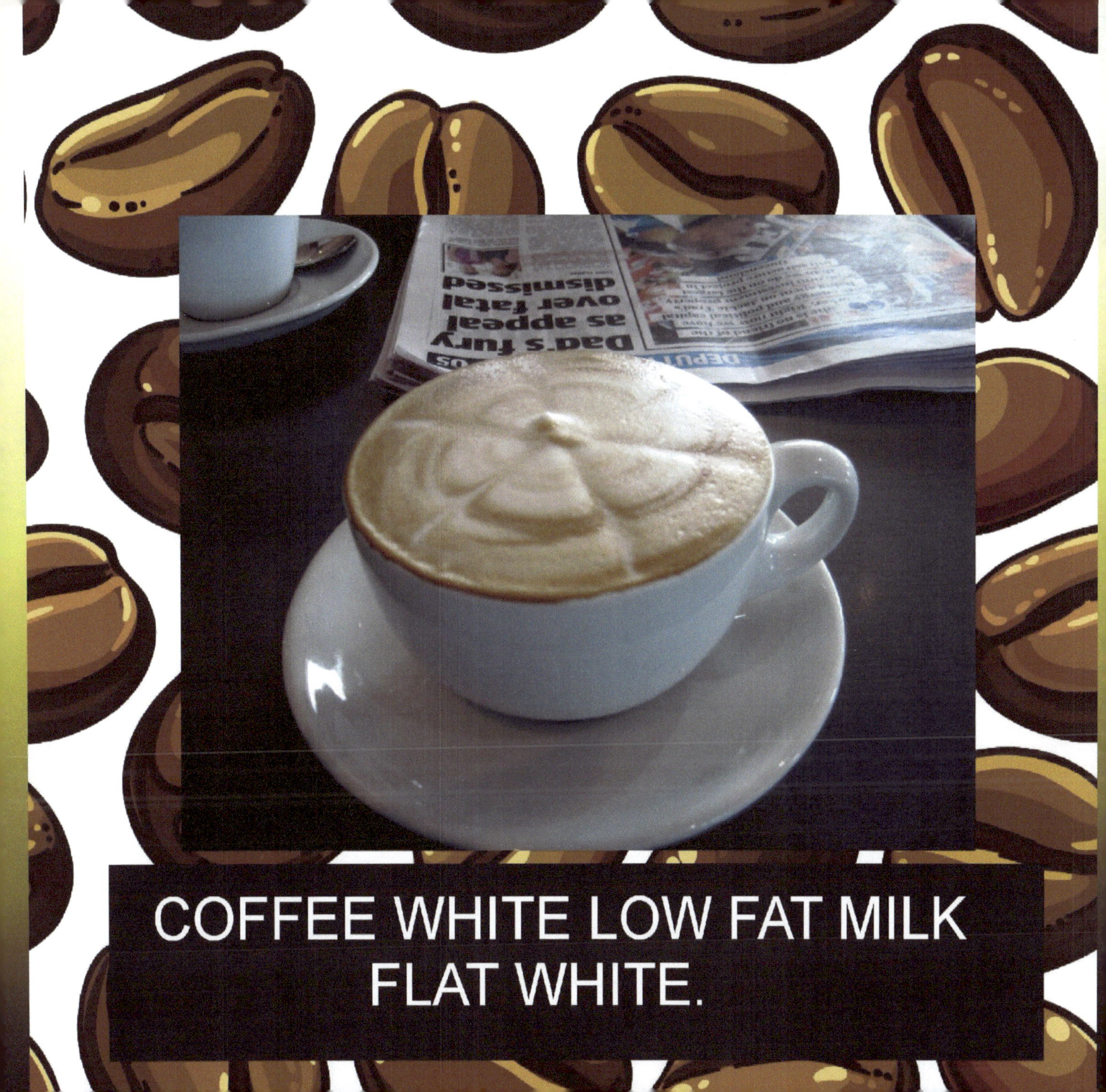

COFFEE WHITE LOW FAT MILK
FLAT WHITE.

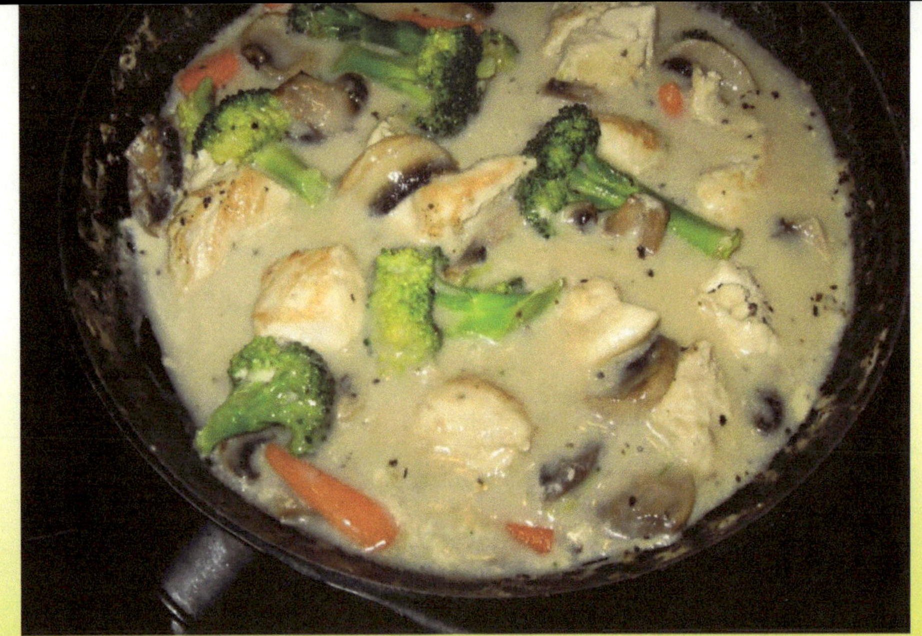

Chicken tenferloins 4 pieces (serves 2)
2 med carrots cut Cook chicken in stock in
small pan add mushrooms 4 med cut.
Broccoli 1/2 head into small pieces,
chicken stock 2 cups
Add 1.5 cups of low fat milk or Lactose free
Thicken with one teaspoon arrowroot
 in water add.
Serve with steamed rice.
Creamy mornay sauce.

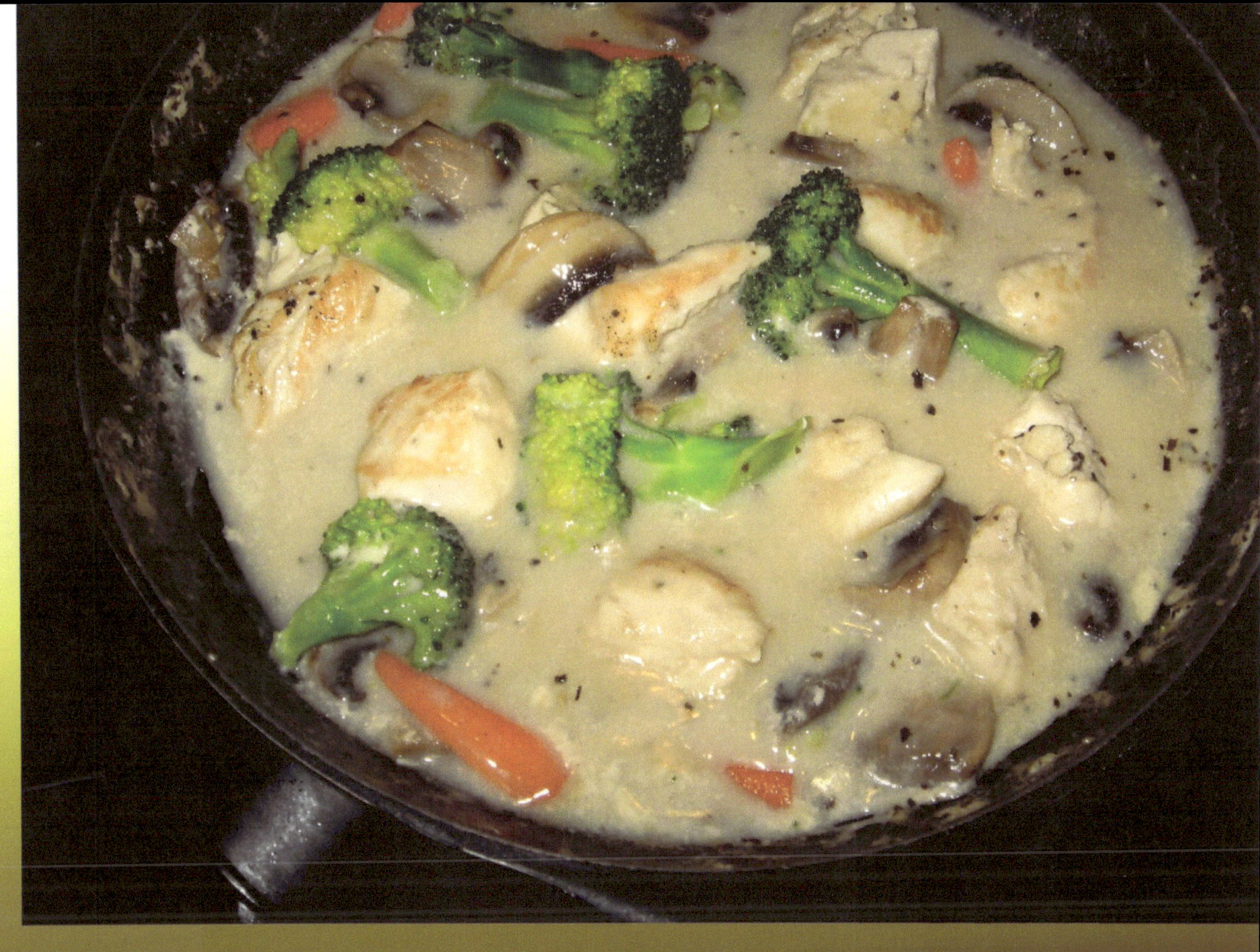

Chicken mornay with mushrooms stir fry.

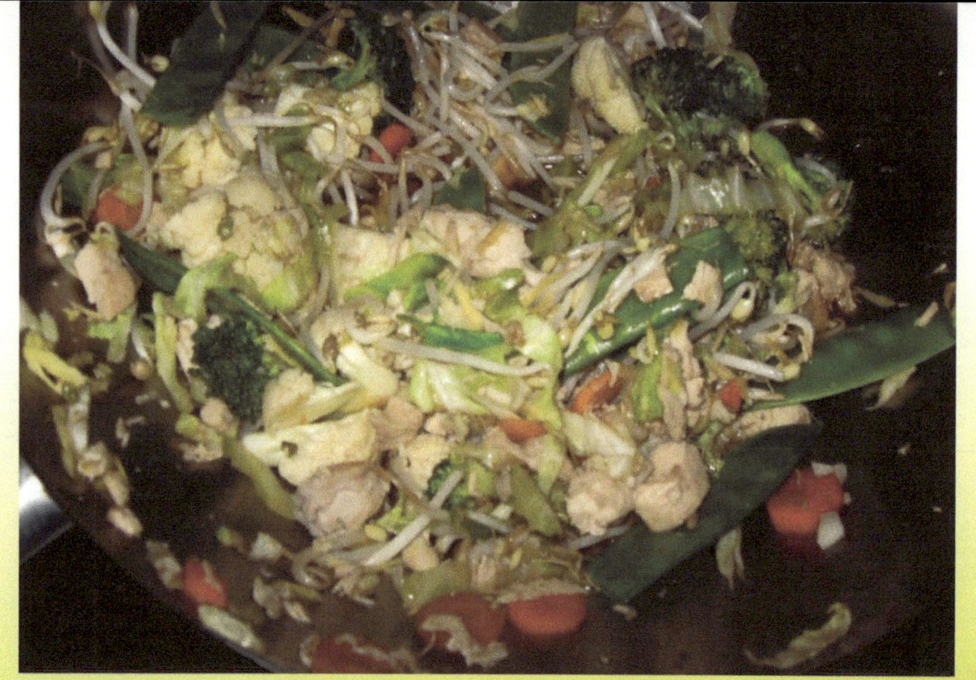

2 pieces (serves 2) salmon cooked in
coconut water 2 med carrots in wheels
small pan add cauliflower pieces .
1.5 cups coconut water , 1 cup bean sprouts
fresh, 8 snow peas in last two minutes
Serve some juice
        Serve with steamed rice.

Salmon in coconut water with stir fry vegs

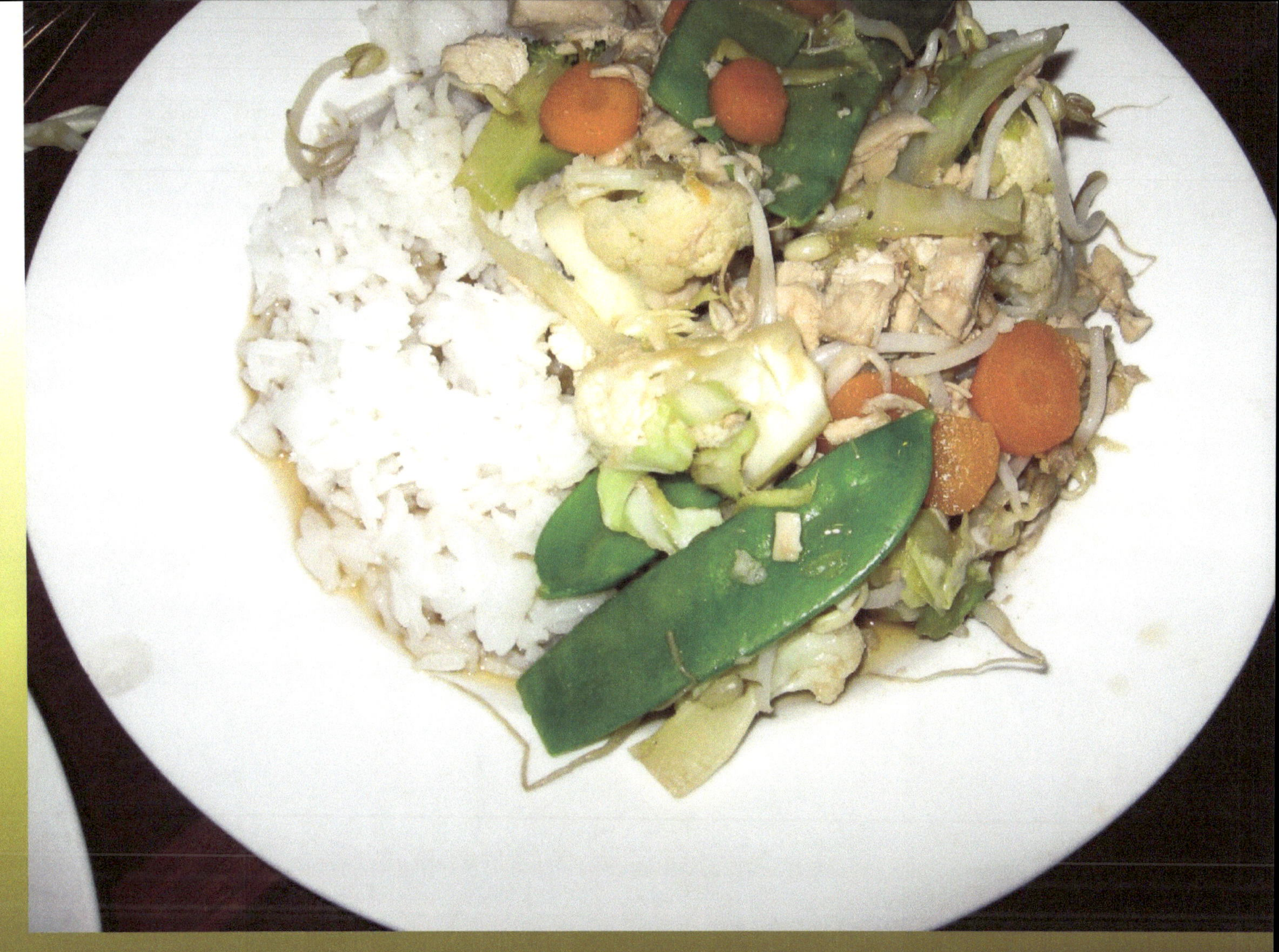

Salmon cooked in coconut water with stir fry vegetables.

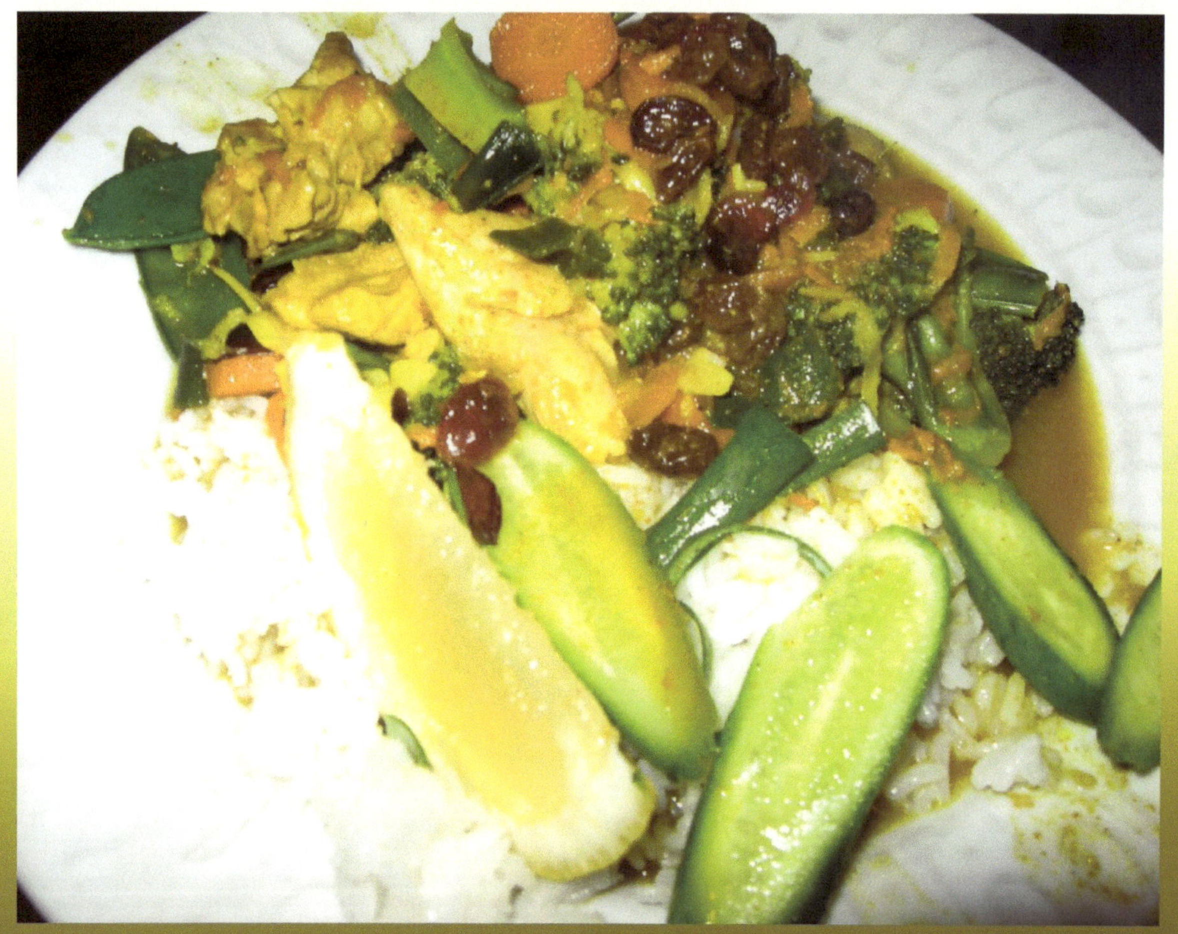

Four pieces of chicken tenderloin cook in small fry pan. Canberries, raisons , snow peas carrots cut into straws,Clive of India one tablespoon , chicken stock serve on rice with cucumber and lemon.

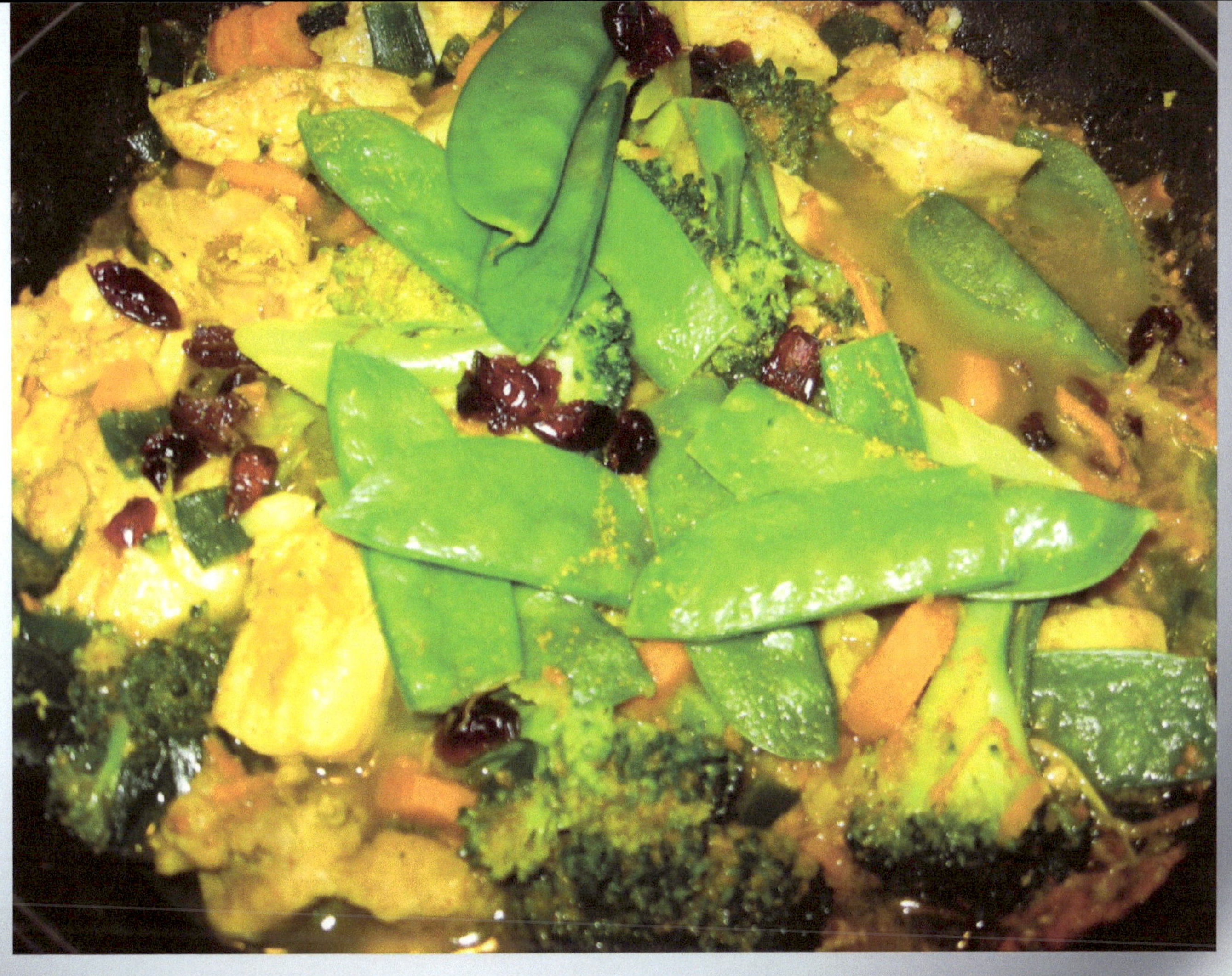

CHICKEN CURRY, CRANBERRIES STIR FRY.

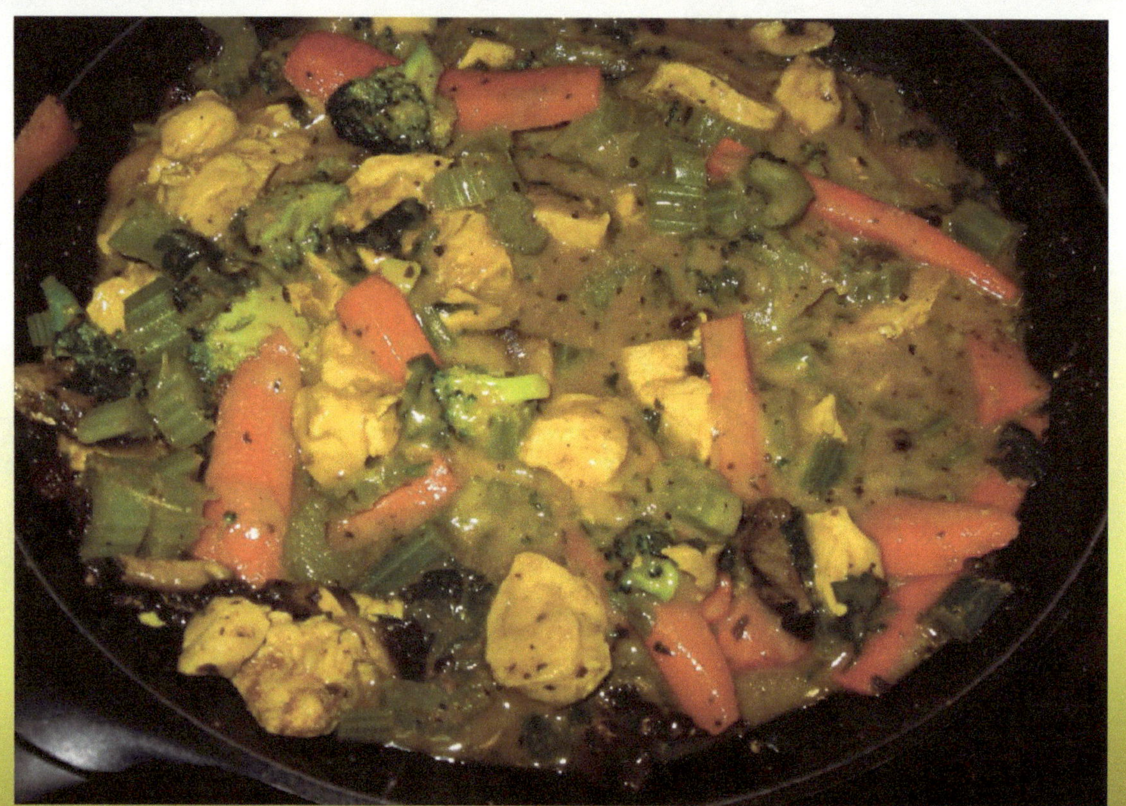

Chicken tenferloins 4 pieces (serves 2)
2 med carrots cut
mushrooms cut 4 med
2 sticks celery incl leaves
Broccoli, cauliflower , Clive of India curry
powder, chicken stock 2 cups
Thicken with arrowroot one spoonful in water
 add. Serve with steamed rice.

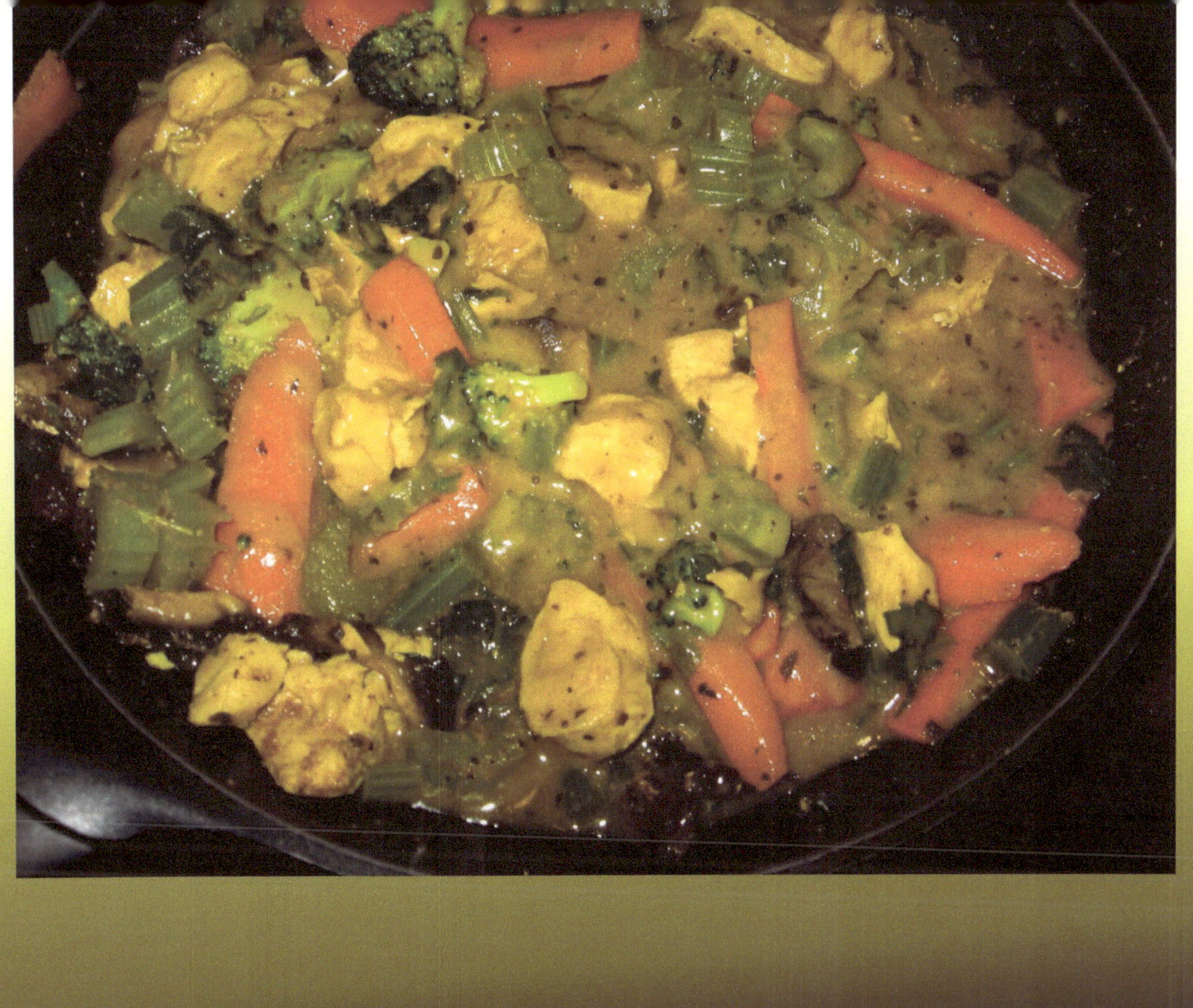

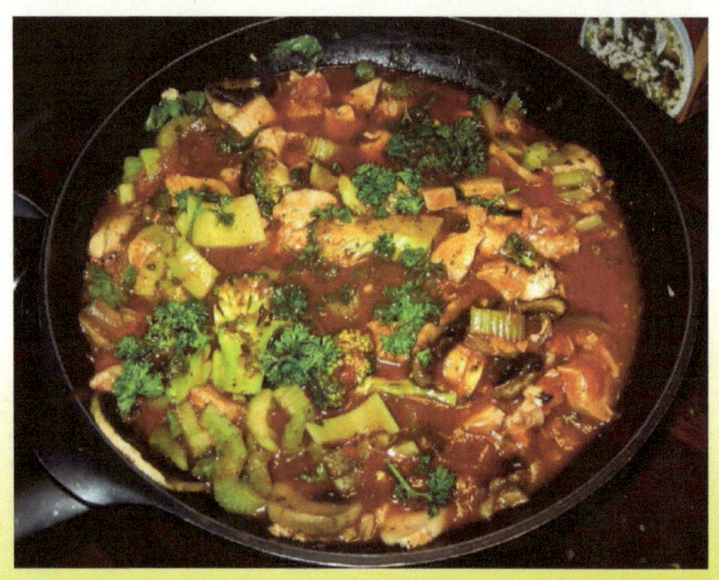

4 pieces (serves 2) chicken cooked in chicken stock, one small tin tomato paste
 2 med carrots in small pan add celery pieces , parsley finely chopped.
 Serve with steamed rice.

Chicken , tomato and garlic.

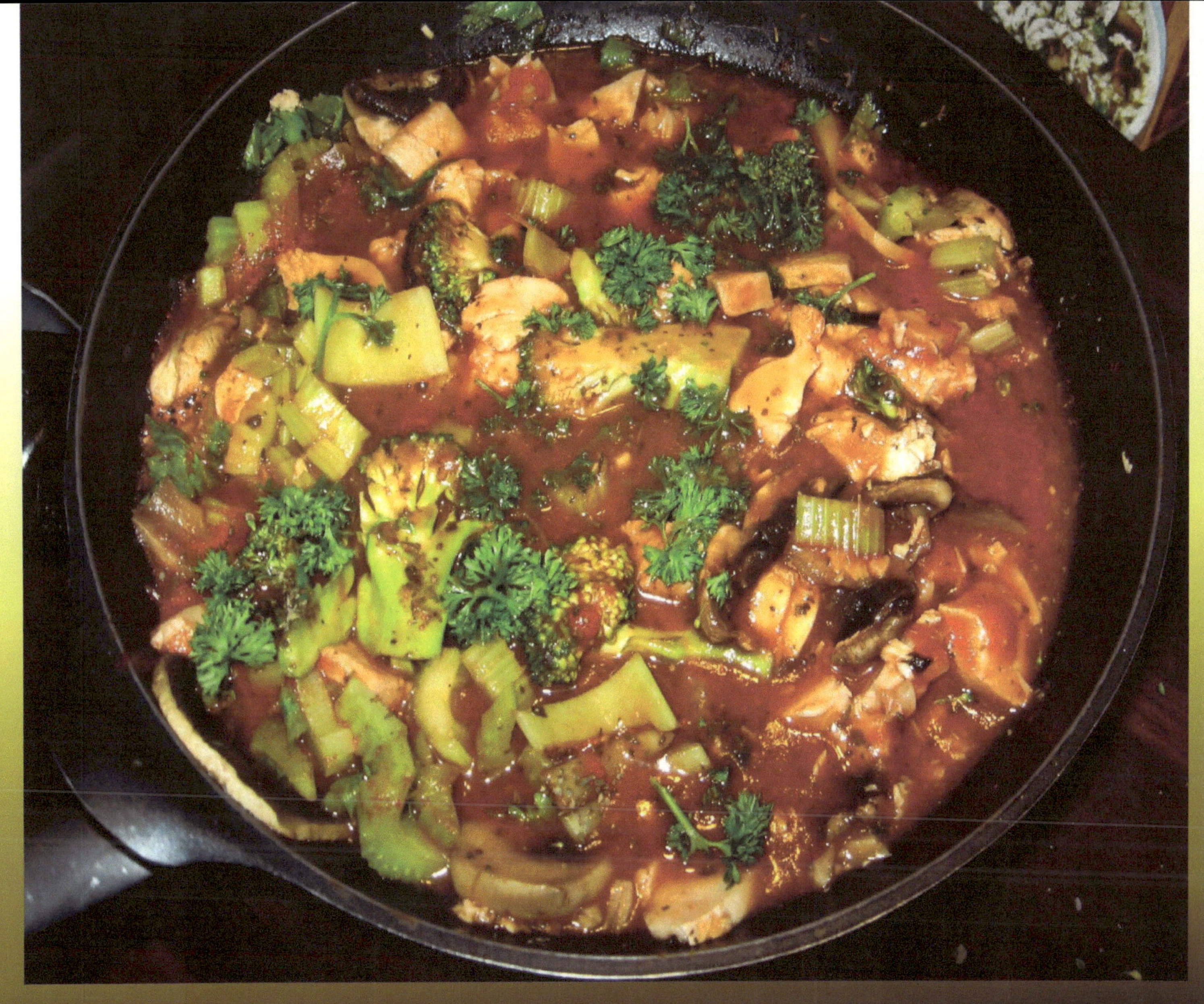

Chicken Medi, tomato garlic

MANDARINE SALAD

Lettuce, baby spinich leaves
tomato cut, red onion sliced thinly,
small mandarine, pumpkin seeds.
Advocado if you want
Balsamic vinegar.
Serve with fish or chicken that is steamed
or grilled.
No baked chicken it will upset
the pancreas.

MANDARINE SALAD

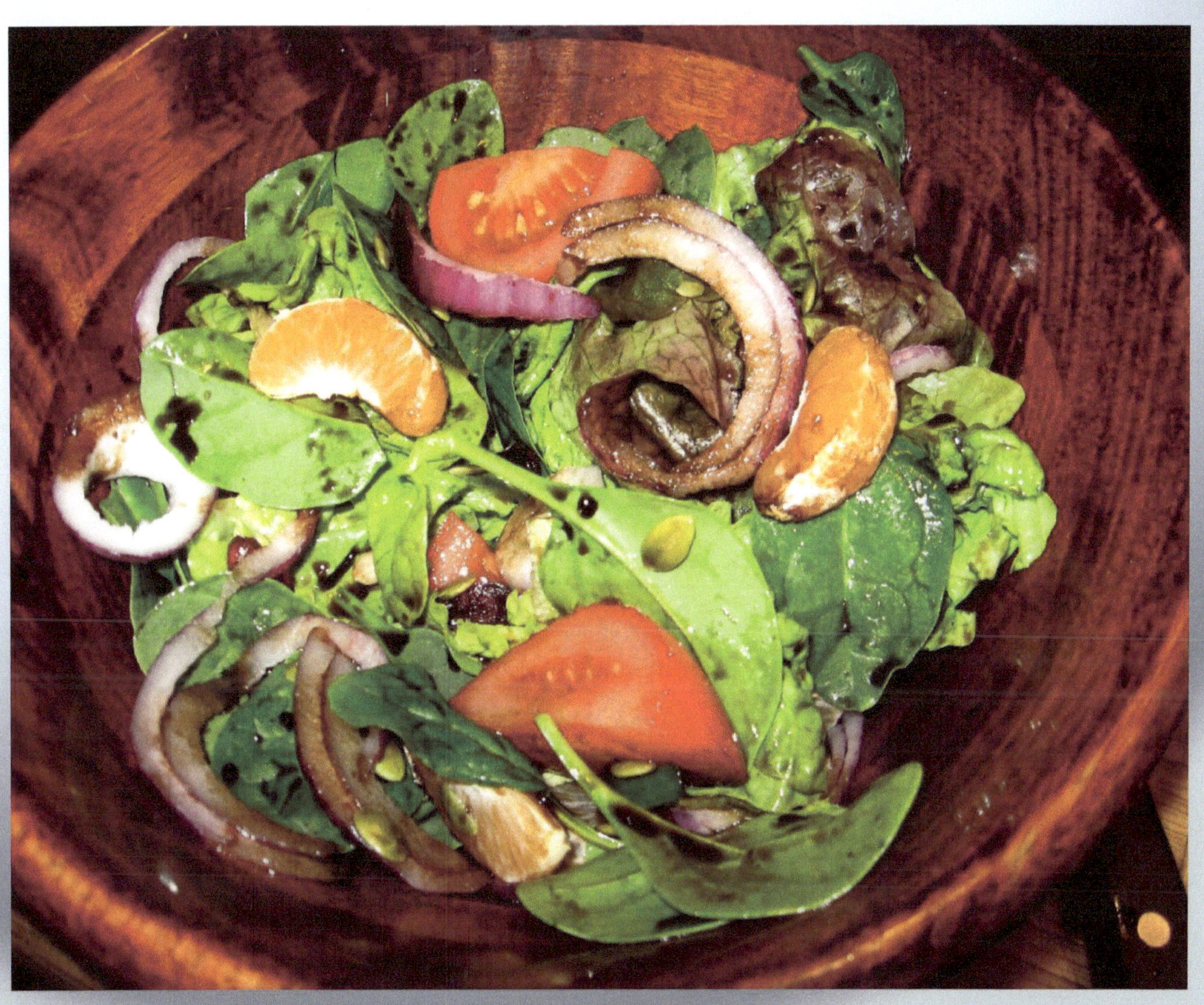

Casserol chicken & prunes.

Casserol dish for microwave
2 cups low fat milk
2 cups cooked chicken breast no skin
8 prunes, 12 cashews , 2 teaspoons
cranberries , one teaspoon arrowroot mixed
in 1/2 cup chicken stock. Sprinkle of basil.
add 1/2 cup frozen peas cook for
10 minutes in microwave.
Serve with steamed carrots and
cut Broccalli.

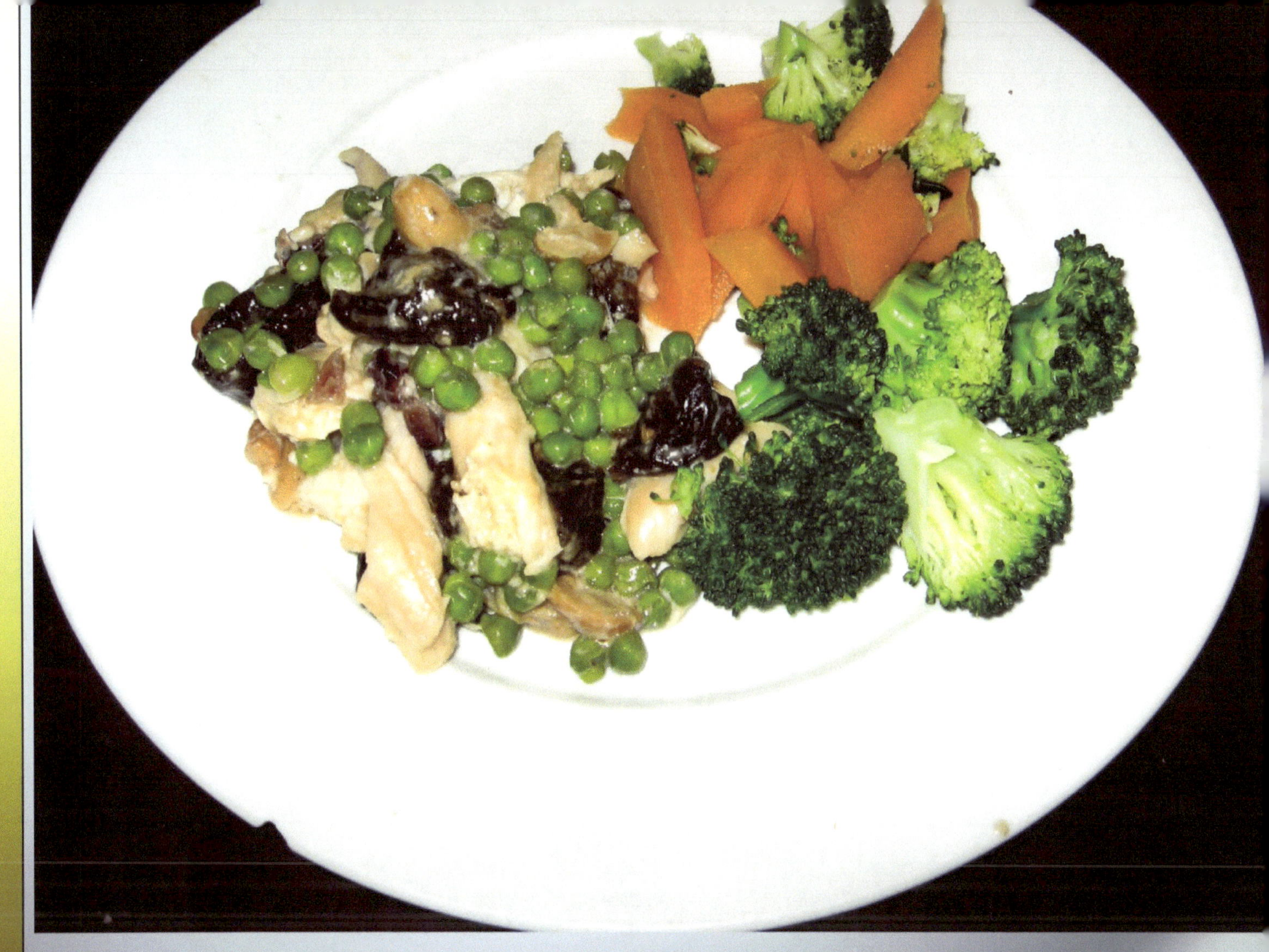

Casserol
chicken &
prunes.

Blueberry and Strawberry Frappe.

one cup almond milk low fat
1/3 cup frozen blueberries
four large strawberries

Blend together in blender
serve with strawberry
garnish.

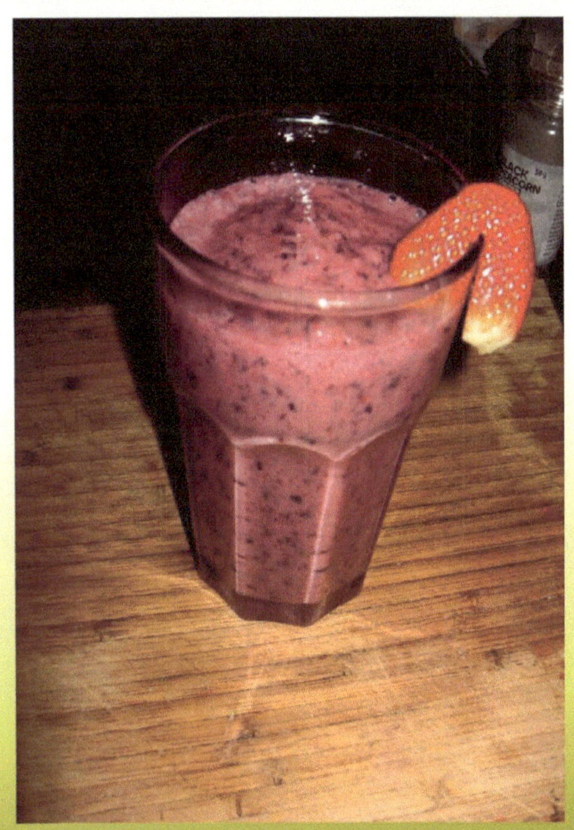

Blueberry & strawberry Frappe

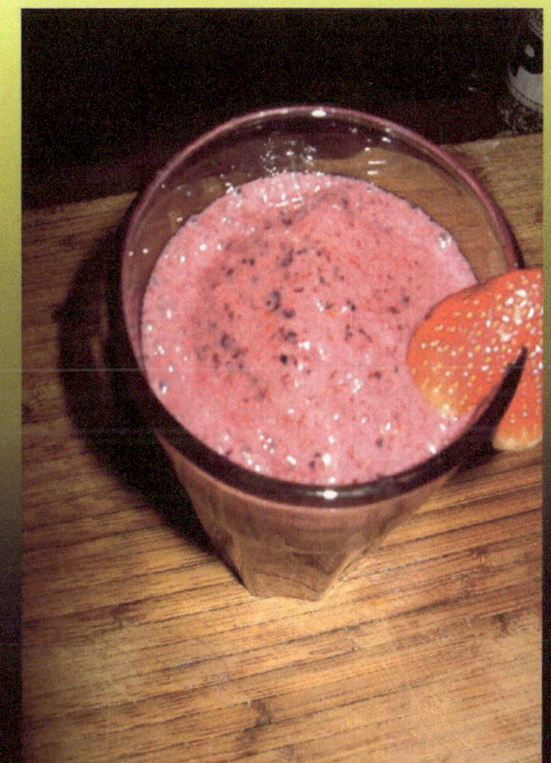

Red salmon cooked in coconut water.

Red salmon cook in 1/2" coconut water
in small electric frypan.

Sweet potato mashed no additives.

Cauliflower with green beans steamed

A simple nutricious meal.

Add lemon slice.

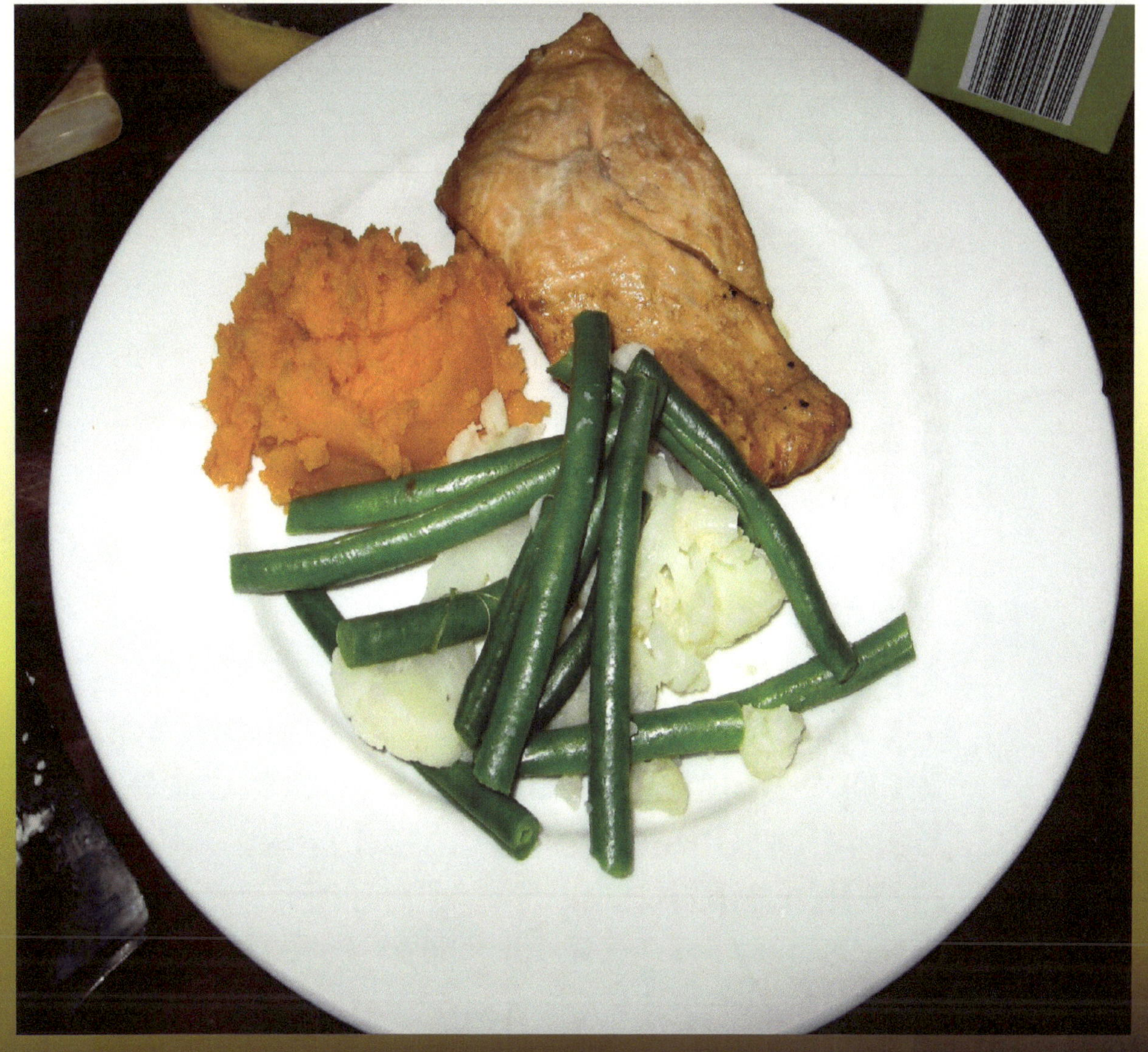

Red salmon cooked in coconut water.

Thai red chicken

SERVES 2

3 Jalapenos (small mild chilli)
4 pieces of chicken tenderloins
1/2 head broccili, 1/3 cup shallots
1/3 cup sliced finely celery
1 tablespoon Thai Red curry paste
1 cup champiogions button mushrooms
2 cups chicken broth (no addiditives)
Serve on Jasmine steamed rice.
COOK CHICKE IN SMALL PIECES IN
CHICKEN STOCK IN SMALL FRYPAN
ADD Thai red curry and mushrooms ,
Jalapenos cut finely add broccili last two
minutes before serving.

Red Thai Curry Chicken

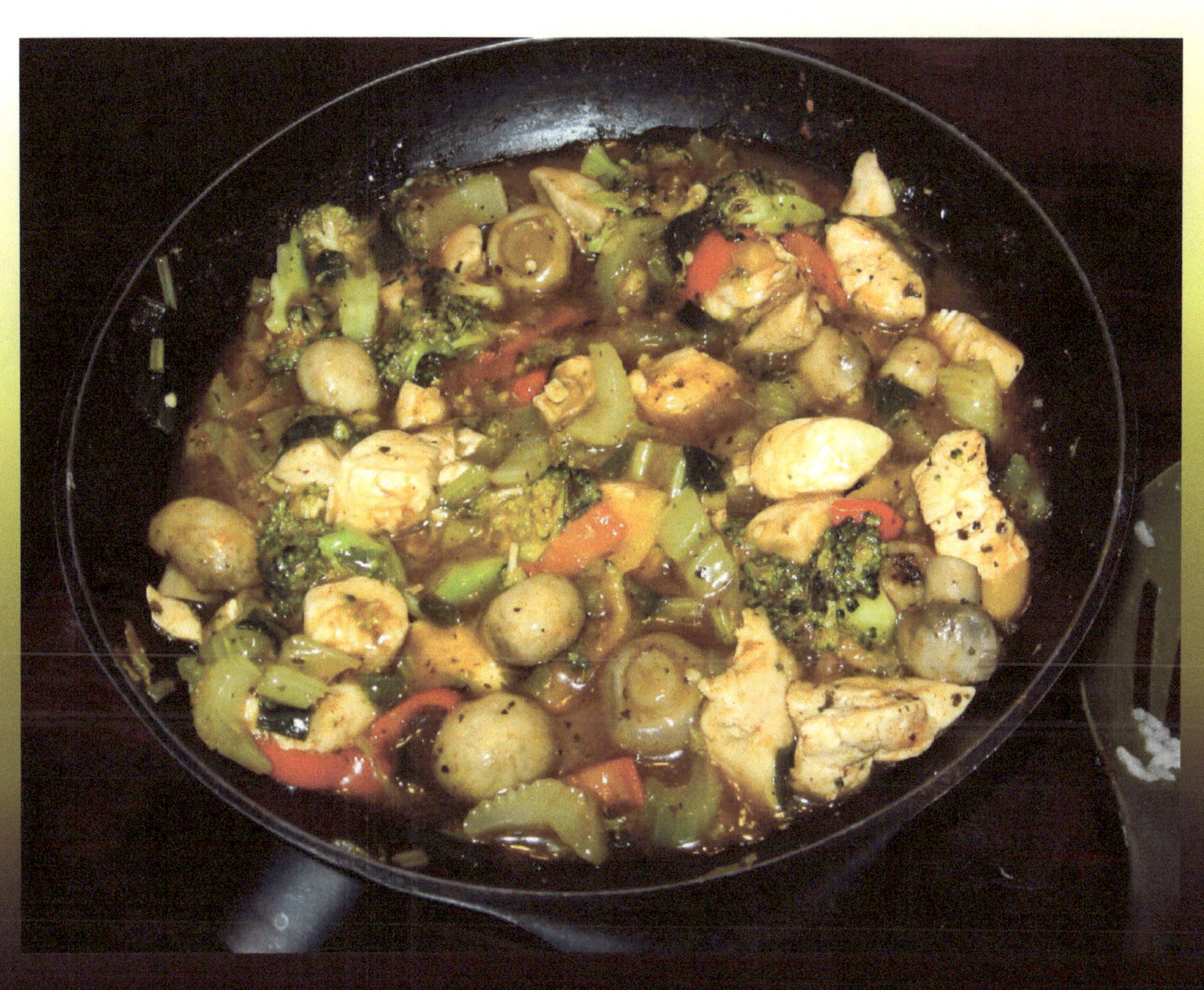

Tropical salad serve with fish

One cup of baby spinich
leaves
one orange cut into small
squares
One half cup of baby beetroot tinned no sugar
pumpkin seed two table spoons
squeeze half a lemon
One tree ripened tomato
one red onion sliced finley
drizzle Balsamic vinegar over and serve.

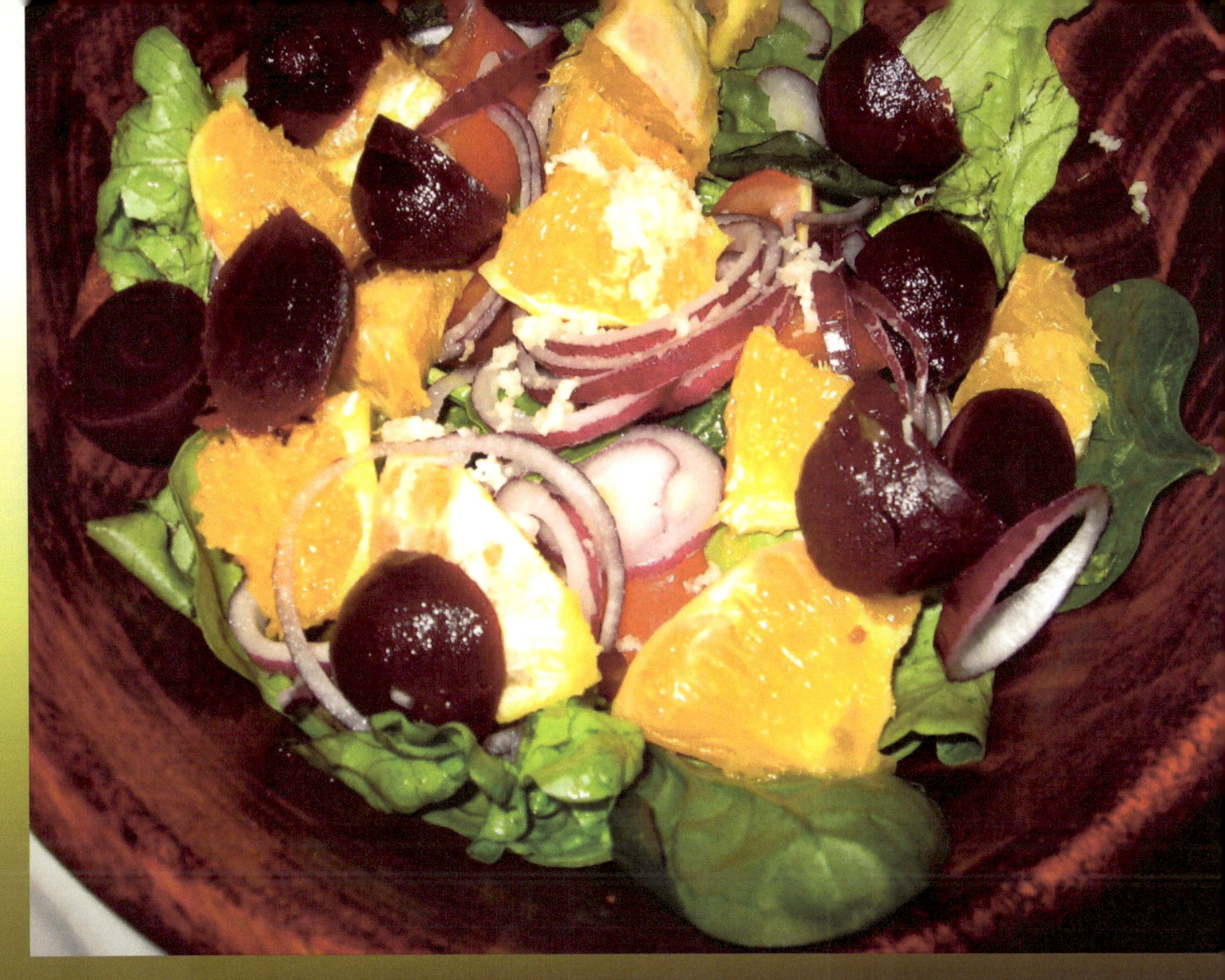

Tropical salad serve with fish

Tuna & Sweetcorn Mornay

One tin sweet corn
one tin Tuna
one pint of milk low fat skim
two tablespoons corn flour mix with portion
of milk. Basil sprinkle on top
Shallots chopped finely
Stir all the time until sauce thickens
medium heat in small omelette pan

SERVE ON STEAMED RICE.

Tuna & Sweetcorn Mornay

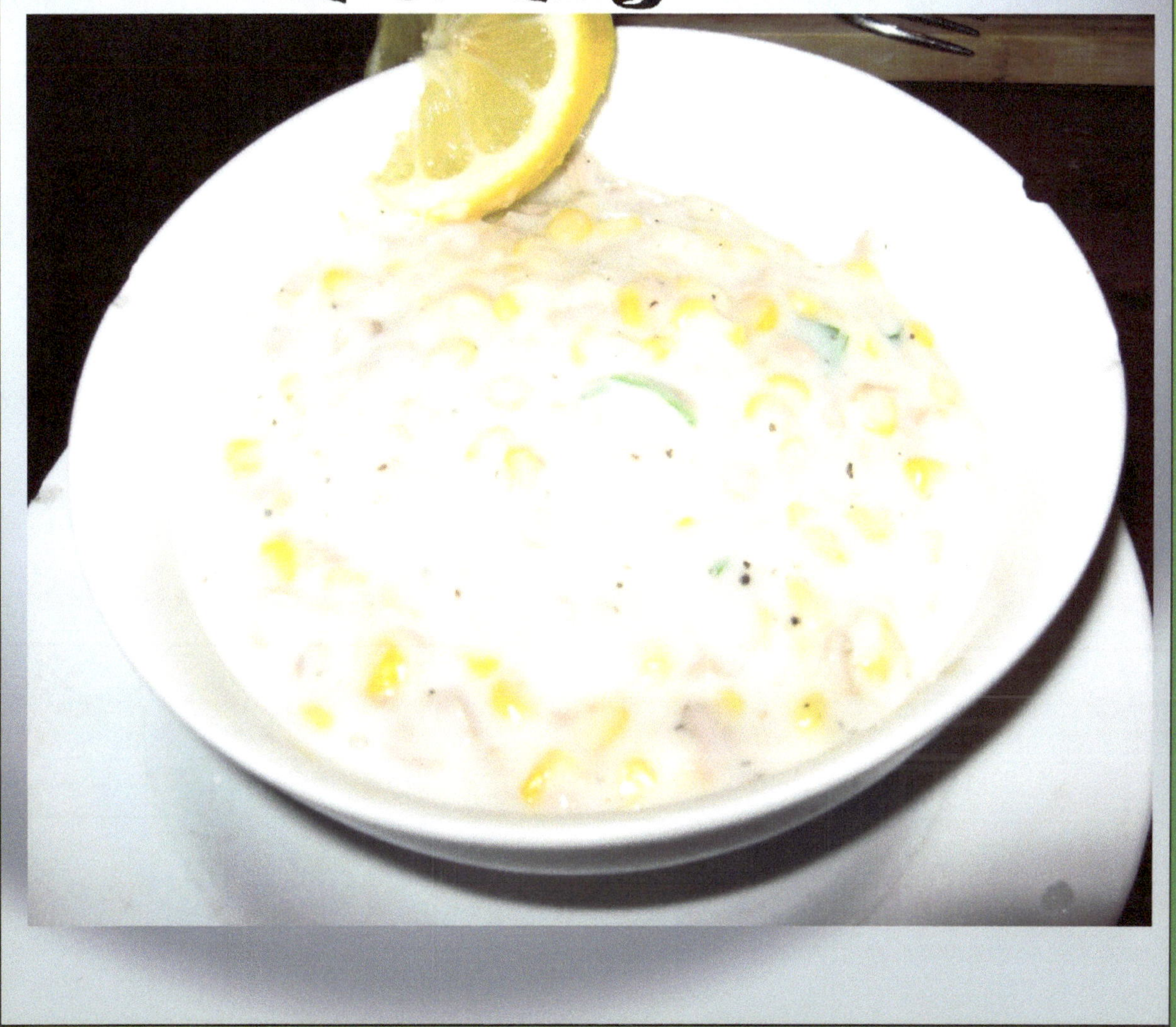

Health Statement.

I was diagnosed as having an accute inflamed pancreas.
The doctor put me on a diet.
NO MEAT, BACON, NO OIL OF ANY TYPE
NO BUTTER OR MARGARINE, NO ROASTS
NO FULL CREAM DAIRY FOODS ONLY NON
FAT , NO PASTA, NO PRESERVES , NO
SUGAR. 3 PIECES OF FRUIT PER DAY,
VEGETABLES, FISH AND CHICKEN
COOKED IN COCONUT WATER or chicken
stock. I was devasted at first.
I was a sous chef so I developed some
tasty recipes keeping withing those guide
lines I hope you enjoy them as much as
I do.

STRAWBERRY FRAPPE'

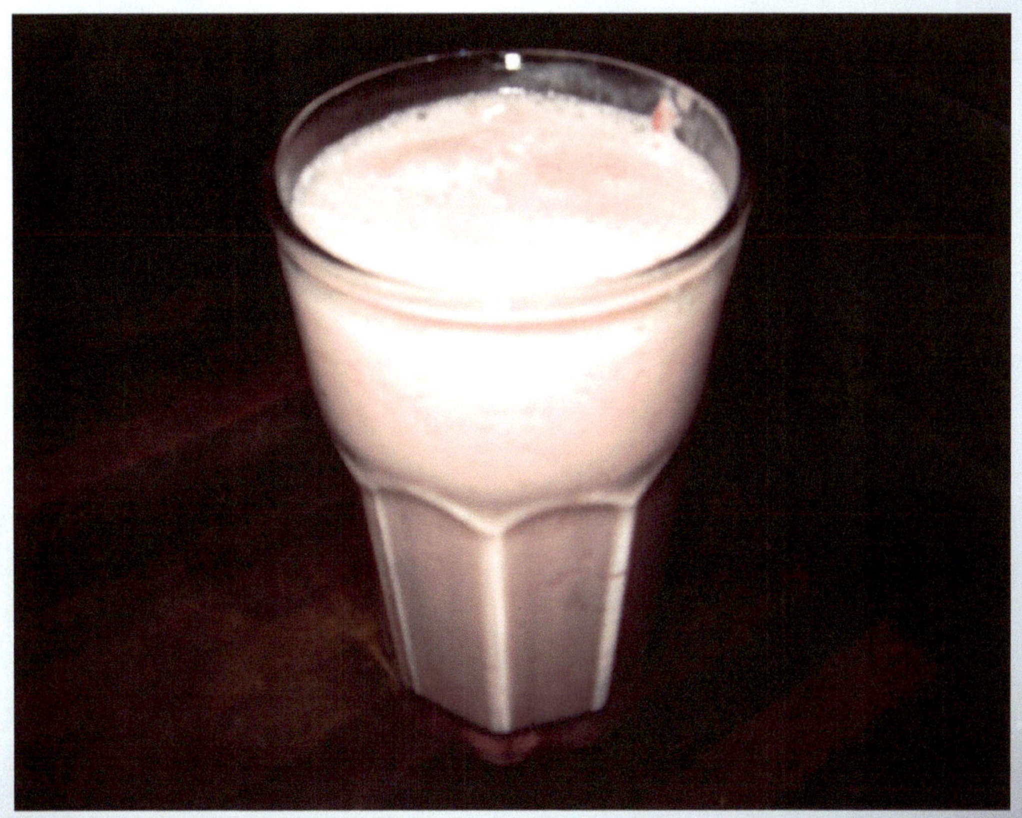

6 strawberries
1.5 cups almond milk
Mix in Blender.

Coconut chicken

One and a half cups chicken stock
4 pieces chicken tenderloin skinned
1/2 tin light coconut milk
snow peas carrots
Champignons one cup small button mushrooms.
One desertsoopful Thai Green curry paste.

Cook mushrooms chicken and carrots, curry
 paste. Add 1/2 tin coconut milk light,
add snow peas
serve 3 minutes later

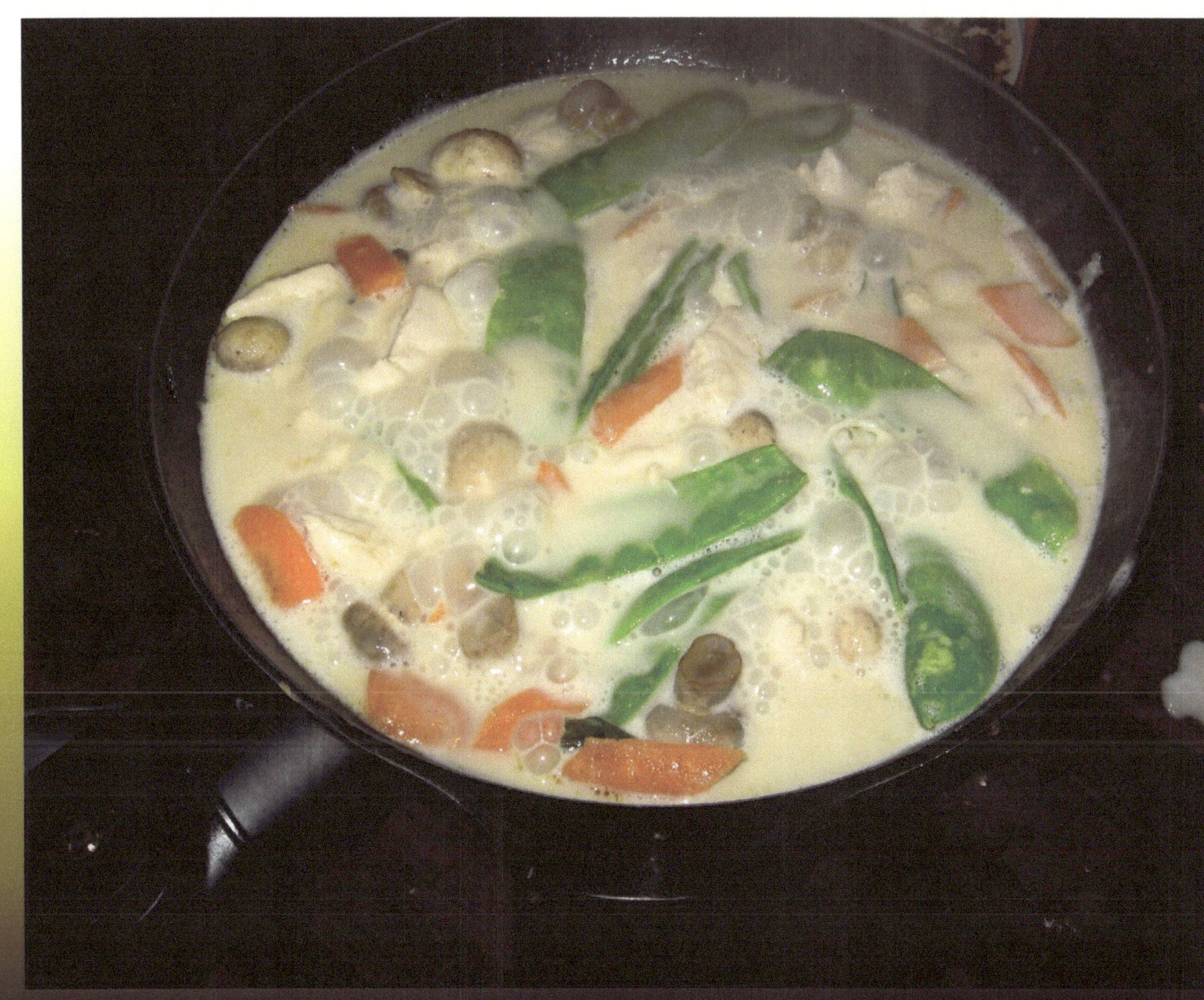

Coconut chicken

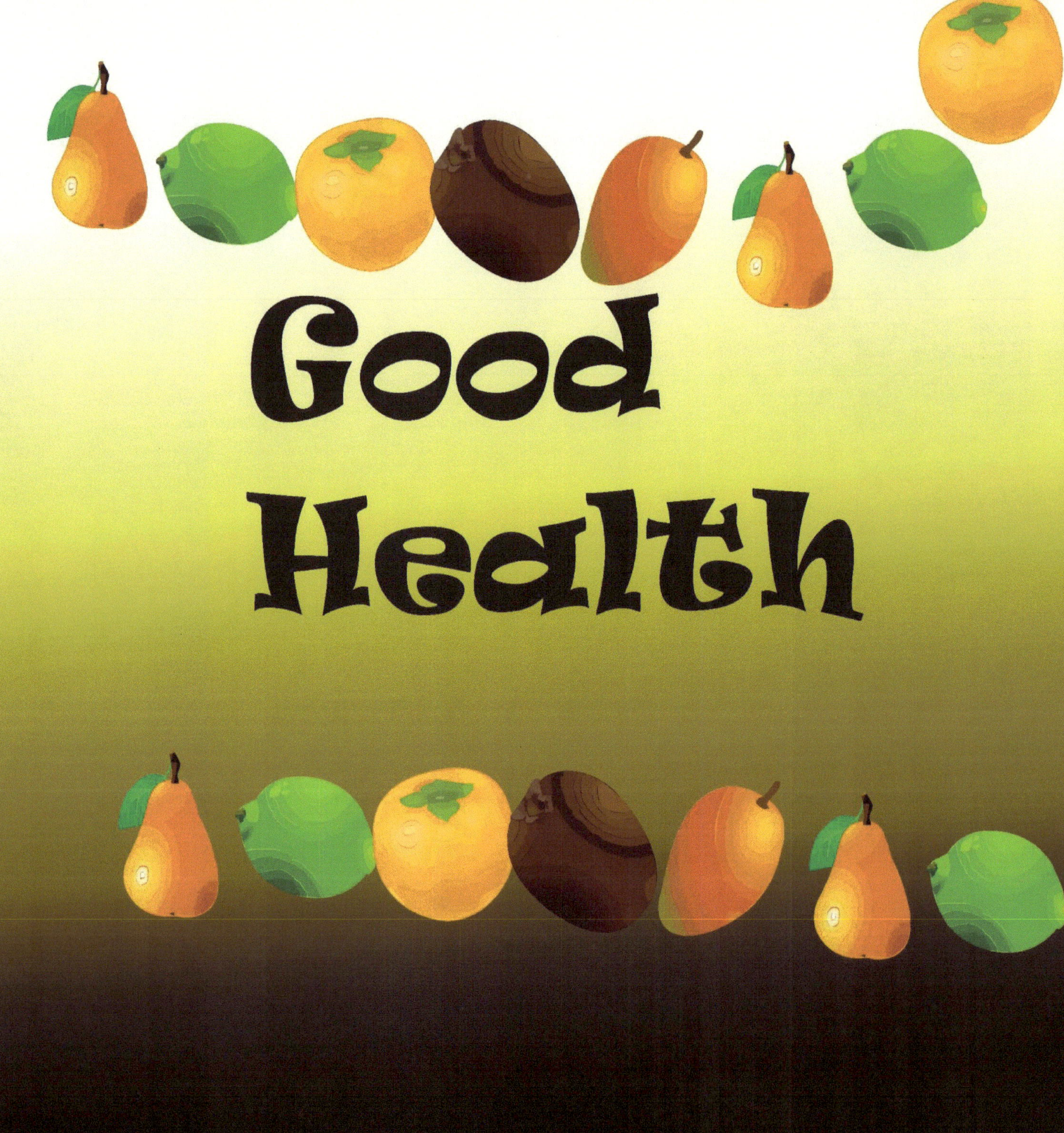
Good
Health